56 All Natural Juice Recipes to Help Cure Urinary Tract Infections:

Quickly Improve Your Condition without Medical Treatments

By

Joe Correa CSN

COPYRIGHT

This publication is designed to provide accurate and authoritative information in regard to the subject matter covered. It is sold with the understanding that neither the author nor the publisher is engaged in rendering medical advice. If medical advice or assistance is needed, consult with a doctor. This book is considered a guide and should not be used in any way detrimental to your health. Consult with a physician before starting this nutritional plan to make sure it's right for you.

ACKNOWLEDGEMENTS

This book is dedicated to my friends and family that have had mild or serious illnesses so that you may find a solution and make the necessary changes in your life.

56 All Natural Juice Recipes to Help Cure Urinary Tract Infections:

Quickly Improve Your Condition without Medical Treatments

By

Joe Correa CSN

CONTENTS

ABOUT THE AUTHOR

After years of Research, I honestly believe in the positive effects that proper nutrition can have over the body and mind. My knowledge and experience has helped me live healthier throughout the years and which I have shared with family and friends. The more you know about eating and drinking healthier, the sooner you will want to change your life and eating habits.

Nutrition is a key part in the process of being healthy and living longer so get started today. The first step is the most important and the most significant.

INTRODUCTION

56 All Natural Juice Recipes to Help Cure Urinary Tract Infections: Quickly Improve Your Condition without Medical Treatments

By Joe Correa CSN

A urinary infection is a group of rather common infections of any part of the urinary tract – kidneys, ureters, bladder, and urethra. These infections are caused by different microbes (mostly bacteria) that overcome the body's ability to defend itself. This condition leads to more frequent urge to urinate followed by a painful and burning sensation and/or strong smelling urine. Studies show that women are more likely to suffer from urinary infections (with the risk of over 50%) at least once in their life with many cases of repeated infections.

Most urinary infections are caused by bacteria Escherichia coli which can be found in the digestive tract and Chlamydia that attacks urethra. In general, everybody can develop some form of urinary infection. However, there are some risk factors that increase the chances of developing repeated urinary infections. These factors include:

- Improper body hygiene
- Diabetes
- Pregnancy
- Urinary catheter
- Blocked urine flow
- Kidney diseases
- Repeated use of antibiotics which affect the natural microflora
- Weakened immune system

Luckily, most urinary infections are easily curable with antibiotics or antimicrobials. In healthy people (with a normal urinary tract) suffering from some form of urinary infection, the treatment takes about 2-3 days. People whose organisms are weakened by some other disease or condition will most likely get more complicated urinary tract infections and their treatment can take between 7-14 days. Pregnant women, older people, and patients suffering from cancer, diabetes, or some other medical problems should be hospitalized until the infection is completely healed.

Having to deal with urinary infections can be quite unpleasant and can disrupt your everyday life and work. Just like with every other health condition, it's better to prevent these infections from happening in the first place.

For this reason, I have created a wonderful collection of juice recipes that will help you heal any urinary infection. Use these recipes to fix your problem naturally and boost your immune system thus preventing infections in the future.

Enjoy them all and try them during different times of the day. Early morning, when you wake up, is the ideal time for one of these juices.

COMMITMENT

In order to improve my condition, I *(your name)*, commit to eating more of these foods on a daily basis and to exercise at least 30 minutes daily:

- Berries (especially blueberries), peaches, cherries, apples, apricots, oranges, lemon juice, grapefruit, tangerines, mandarins, pears, etc.
- Broccoli, spinach, collard greens, sweet potatoes, avocado, artichoke, baby corn, carrots, celery, cauliflower, onions, etc.
- Whole grains, steel-cut oats, oatmeal, quinoa, barley, etc.
- Black beans, red bean beans, garbanzo beans, lentils, etc.
- Nuts and seeds including: walnuts, cashews, flaxseeds, sesame seeds, etc.
- Fish
- 8 – 10 glasses of water

Sign here

X_____

56 ALL NATURAL JUICE RECIPES TO HELP CURE URINARY TRACT INFECTIONS

1.   Raspberry Cranberry Juice

Ingredients:

1 cup of fresh blueberries

1 cup of fresh raspberries

1 cup of fresh cranberries

1 large lemon, peeled

1 cup of watermelon, seeded

1 tbsp of maple syrup

Preparation:

Combine raspberries, cranberries, and blueberries in a large colander. Rinse under cold running water. Drain and set aside.

Peel the lemon and cut lengthwise in half. Set aside.

Cut the watermelon lengthwise. For one cup, you will need about 1 large wedge. Peel and cut into chunks.

Remove the seeds and set aside. Reserve the rest of the melon for some other juices.

Now, process berries, lemon and watermelon in a juicer.

Transfer to serving glasses and stir in the maple syrup.

Add some ice cubes before serving.

Enjoy!

Nutrition information per serving: Kcal: 230, Protein: 4.1g, Carbs: 53.1g, Fats: 1.7g

2.   Apple Celery Juice

Ingredients:

1 medium-sized green apple, cored

3-4 large celery stalks

2 large beets, trimmed

3 large carrots, sliced

1 large lemon, peeled

¼ tsp ginger, ground

A handful of fresh kale, torn

Preparation:

Wash the apple and remove the core. Cut into bite-sized pieces and set aside.

Wash the celery stalks and chop into small pieces. Set aside.

Wash the beets and trim off the green parts. Cut into bite-sized pieces and set aside.

Wash the carrots and cut into thick slices. Set aside.

Peel the lemon and cut lengthwise in half. Set aside.

Wash the kale thoroughly and torn with hands. Set aside.

Now, combine apple, celery, kale, beets, carrots, and lemon in a juicer. Process until juiced.

Transfer to serving glasses and stir in the ginger. Add some ice and serve immediately.

Nutrition information per serving: Kcal: 136, Protein: 6.1g, Carbs: 39g, Fats: 1.2g

3.   Radish Melon Juice

Ingredients:

2 medium-sized radishes

1 medium-sized honeydew melon

1 cup of pomegranate seeds

1 cup of watermelon, seeded

1 cup of beets, trimmed

2 tsp maple syrup

Preparation:

Rinse the beets and radishes and trim off the green parts. Chop into small pieces and set aside.

Cut the honeydew melon lengthwise in half. Scoop out the seeds using a spoon. Cut into large wedges and peel them. Now, cut into small chunks and place in a bowl. Set aside.

Cut the top of the pomegranate fruit using a sharp knife. Slice down to each of the white membranes inside of the fruit. Pop the seeds into a measuring cup and set aside.

Cut the watermelon lengthwise. For one cup, you will need about 1 large wedge. Peel and cut into chunks. Remove the seeds and set aside. Reserve the rest of the melon for some other juices.

Now, combine radishes, honeydew melon, pomegranate seeds, watermelon, and beets in a juicer.

Transfer to serving glasses and stir in the maple syrup.

Add some ice and serve.

Nutrition information per serving: Kcal: 167, Protein: 13.1g, Carbs: 45.9g, Fats: 1.5g

4.   Blueberry Apple Juice

Ingredients:

1 cup of blueberries

1 medium-sized apple, cored

1 cup of beets, trimmed

2 small carrots, sliced

1 large lemon, peeled

2 oz water

Preparation:

Rinse the blueberries under cold running water. Drain and set aside.

Wash the apple and remove the core. Cut into small pieces and set aside.

Wash the beets and trim off the green parts. Cut into bite-sized pieces and set aside.

Wash the carrots and cut into thick slices. Set aside.

Peel the lemon and cut lengthwise in half. Set aside.

Now, combine blueberries, apple, beets, carrots, and lemon in a juicer. Process until juiced.

Transfer to serving glasses and stir in the coconut water. Garnish with mint and refrigerate before serving.

Enjoy!

Nutrition information per serving: Kcal: 240, Protein: 5.6g, Carbs: 74.1g, Fats: 1.5g

5. Lime Cinnamon Juice

Ingredients:

2 large limes, peeled

¼ tsp of cinnamon, ground

3 large oranges, peeled

2 large lemons, peeled

2 tsp agave nectar

2 oz water

Preparation:

Peel the lemons and limes and cut lengthwise in half. Set aside.

Peel the oranges and divide into wedges. Set aside.

Now, combine limes, oranges, and lemons in a juicer.

Transfer to serving glasses and stir in the cinnamon, agave, and water.

Add few ice cubes and serve immediately.

Nutrition information per serving: Kcal: 246, Protein: 6.8g, Carbs: 83.1g, Fats: 1.1g

6.   Celery Leek Juice

Ingredients:

1 cup fresh celery

3 large leeks, chopped

2 cups beet greens, trimmed

1 cup fresh kale, torn

1 large cucumber, sliced

¼ tsp ginger powder

Preparation:

Wash the beet greens and kale thoroughly and torn with hands. Set aside.

Peel the onion and cut in half. Cut one slice and reserve the rest for some other juice or meal.

Wash the celery and leek. Cut into small pieces and set aside.

Wash the cucumber and cut into thick slices. Set aside.

Now, combine celery, leek, beet greens, cucumber, and ginger in a juicer. Process until juiced.

Transfer to serving glasses and refrigerate for 5 minutes before serving.

Nutritional information per serving: Kcal: 230, Protein: 11.5g, Carbs: 63.2g, Fats: 2.1g

7.   Strawberry Apple Juice

Ingredients:

1 cup fresh strawberries, chopped

1 medium-sized Red Delicious apple, cored

1 cup fresh blackberries

1 cup green grapes

2 oz coconut water

Preparation:

Combine strawberries and blackberries in a colander. Wash under cold running water and set aside.

Wash the apple and remove the core. Cut into bite-sized pieces and set aside.

Rinse the grapes and remove the stems. Set aside.

Now, combine strawberries, apple, blackberries, and grapes in a juicer. Process until juiced. Transfer to serving glasses and stir in the coconut water.

Add some ice cubes before serving.

Nutritional information per serving: Kcal: 201, Protein: 4.3g, Carbs: 63.4g, Fats: 1.7g

8.   Cucumber Cantaloupe Juice

Ingredients:

1 large cucumber

1 cup cantaloupe, cubed

1 large honeydew melon wedge

1 cup watermelon, seeded

1 tbsp agave nectar

Preparation:

Wash the cucumber and cut into thick slices. Set aside.

Cut the cantaloupe in half. Scoop out the seeds and flesh. Cut two wedges and peel them. Chop into chunks and set aside. Reserve the rest of the cantaloupe in a refrigerator.

Cut the honeydew melon lengthwise in half. Scoop out the seeds using a spoon. Cut one large wedge and peel. Cut into small chunks and place in a bowl. Wrap the rest of the melon in a plastic foil and refrigerate.

Cut the watermelon lengthwise. For one cup, you will need about 1 large wedge. Peel and cut into chunks. Remove the seeds and set aside. Reserve the rest of for some other juices.

Now, combine cucumber, cantaloupe, honeydew melon, and watermelon in a juicer.

Transfer to serving glasses and stir in the agave. Add some ice before serving.

Enjoy!

Nutritional information per serving: Kcal: 201, Protein: 3.4g, Carbs: 57.6g, Fats: 0.8g

9. Lettuce Watermelon Juice

Ingredients:

2 cups red leaf lettuce, shredded

1 cup watermelon, diced

2 cups raspberries

1 cup beets, chopped

¼ cup water

Preparation:

Wash the lettuce thoroughly and torn with hands. Set aside.

Cut the watermelon lengthwise. For one cup, you will need about 1 large wedge. Peel and cut into chunks. Remove the seeds and set aside. Reserve the rest of for some other juices.

Wash the raspberries under cold running water. Drain and set aside.

Wash the beets and trim off the green parts. Cut into small pieces and set aside.

Now, combine lettuce, watermelon, raspberries, and beets in a juicer.

Transfer to serving glasses and stir in the water.

Add some ice and serve immediately.

Nutritional information per serving: Kcal: 157, Protein: 6.8g, Carbs: 55g, Fats: 2.1g

10.   Orange Chard Juice

Ingredients:

2 large oranges, peeled

1 cup Swiss chard, chopped

4 large cucumbers, peeled

3 large carrots, chopped

Preparation:

Peel the oranges and divide into wedges. Set aside.

Rinse the Swiss chard thoroughly under cold running water using a colander. Roughly chop it and set aside.

Wash the cucumbers and carrots. Cut into thick slices and set aside.

Now, combine oranges, Swiss chard, cucumbers, and carrots in a juicer and process until juiced.

Transfer to serving glasses and add some ice cubes.

Enjoy!

Nutritional information per serving: Kcal: 283, Protein: 9g, Carbs: 88.9g, Fats: 1.6g

11.   Squash Pear Juice

Ingredients:

4 cups butternut squash, sliced

1 large pear, cored

1 cup of purple cabbage, shredded

½ cup water

Preparation:

Peel the butternut squash and cut in half. Scoop out the seeds using a spoon. Cut into small chunks and set aside. Reserve the rest in the refrigerator.

Wash the pear and remove the core. Cut into bite-sized pieces and set aside.

Rinse the cabbage thoroughly and shred it. Set aside.

Now, combine butternut squash, pear, and green cabbage in a juicer and process until juiced.

Transfer to serving glasses and stir in the water.

Add some ice and serve immediately.

Nutritional information per serving: Kcal: 192, Protein: 7g, Carbs: 59.9g, Fats: 1.7g

12.   Avocado Celery Juice

Ingredients:

1 cup avocado, sliced

1 cup celery, chopped

1 tbsp fresh mint, finely chopped

1 cup green cabbage, torn

½ cup coconut water, unsweetened

Preparation:

Peel the avocado and cut in half. Remove the pit and cut into chunks. Set aside.

Wash the celery and cut into small pieces. Set aside.

Wash the cabbage thoroughly and torn with hands. Set aside.

Now, combine avocado, celery, and cabbage in a juicer. Process until juiced. Transfer to serving glasses and stir in coconut water and fresh mint.

Add some ice before serving.

Enjoy!

Nutritional information per serving: Kcal: 219, Protein: 4.8g, Carbs: 20.8g, Fats: 21.6g

13.   Orange Grapefruit Juice

Ingredients:

2 large oranges, peeled

1 large grapefruit, peeled

2 cups asparagus, chopped

1 tbsp mint, finely chopped

¼ cup of water

Preparation:

Peel the oranges and grapefruit. Divide into wedges and set aside.

Rinse the asparagus under cold running water. Trim off the woody ends and chop into small pieces. Fill the measuring cups and set aside.

Now, combine asparagus, oranges, and grapefruit in a juicer and process until juiced.

Transfer to serving glasses and stir in the finely chopped mint and water. Add few ice cubes and serve immediately.

Nutritional information per serving: Kcal: 255, Protein: 11.2g, Carbs: 79.8g, Fats: 1.1g

14.   Granny Smith's Juice

Ingredients:

1 cup pineapple, chopped

1 cup sweet cherries, pitted

1 large Honeycrisp apple, cored

2 large kiwis, peeled

Preparation:

Cut the top of a pineapple and peel it using a sharp knife. Cut into small chunks. Reserve the rest of the pineapple in a refrigerator.

Wash the cherries under cold running water. Drain and remove the pits. Set aside.

Wash the apple and remove the core. Cut into bite-sized pieces and set aside.

Peel the kiwis and cut lengthwise in half. Set aside.

Now, combine pineapple, cherries, apple, and kiwis in a juicer and process until juiced.

Transfer to serving glasses and serve immediately.

Nutrition information per serving: Kcal: 287, Protein: 4.2g, Carbs: 84.5g, Fats: 1.2g

15.   Blackberry Banana Juice

Ingredients:

1 cup of blackberries

1 large banana, peeled

1 cup of blueberries

1 tsp maple syrup

½ tsp cinnamon, ground

Preparation:

Combine blackberries and blueberries in a colander. Rinse under cold running water and drain. Set aside.

Peel the banana and chop into chunks. Set aside.

Now, combine berries and banana in a juicer. Process until juiced.

Transfer to serving glasses and stir in the honey and cinnamon.

Add some ice and serve immediately.

Enjoy!

Nutritional information per serving: Kcal: 229, Protein: 4.5g, Carbs: 76.3g, Fats: 1.6g

16.   Blackberry Cucumber Juice

Ingredients:

1 cup of fresh blackberries

1 large cucumber, sliced

1 cup pomegranate seeds

1 whole lime, peeled

A handful of fresh parsley

Preparation:

Rinse the blackberries under cold running water. Drain and set aside.

Wash the cucumber and cut into thick slices. Set aside.

Cut the top of the pomegranate fruit using a sharp knife. Slice down to each of the white membranes inside of the fruit. Pop the seeds into a medium bowl.

Peel the lime and cut in half. Set aside.

Rinse the parsley thoroughly and roughly chop with hands. Set aside.

Now, combine pomegranate seeds, blackberries, cucumber, lime, and parsley in a juicer. Process until juiced.

Transfer to serving glasses and add some ice cubes before serving.

Nutritional information per serving: Kcal: 152, Protein: 8.1g, Carbs: 58.6g, Fats: 2.7g

17.   Parsnip Celery Juice

1 cup parsnips, chopped

1 large celery stalk, chopped

1 whole guava, chopped

2 large grapefruits, peeled

¼ cup water

Preparation:

Wash the parsnips and cut into small slices. Set aside.

Rinse the celery and cut into small pieces. Set aside.

Wash the guava and cut into chunks. If you are using large fruit, reserve the rest for some other recipe in a refrigerator.

Peel the grapefruits and chop into bite-sized pieces.

Now, combine parsnips, celery, guava, grapefruits in a juicer. Process until juiced.

Transfer to serving glasses and add some ice before serving.

Nutritional information per serving: Kcal: 279, Protein: 7.2g, Carbs: 86g, Fats: 1.7g

18.   Apple Goji Juice

Ingredients:

2 small Granny Smith's apples, cored

1 cup goji berries

1 cup fresh cherries, pitted

1 cup beets

3 large tomatoes, peeled

Preparation:

Wash the apples and remove the core. Cut into bite-sized pieces and set aside.

Place the goji berries in a medium bowl and add 1 cup of hot water. Soak for 10 minutes before juicing. Remove the water and set aside.

Wash the beets and trim off the green parts. Cut into small pieces and set aside.

Wash the cherries and remove the pits. Set aside.

Rinse the tomatoes and place in a bowl. Chop into quarters and reserve the juice while cutting.

Now, combine apples, goji berries, beets, cherries, and tomatoes in a juicer.

Transfer to serving glasses and stir in the reserved tomato juice.

Refrigerate for 10 minutes before serving.

Nutritional information per serving: Kcal: 318, Protein: 9.5g, Carbs: 98g, Fats: 2.4g

19.   Cranberry Pineapple Juice

Ingredients:

1 cup cranberries

1 cup pineapple, chunked

1 medium-sized apple, chopped

1 cup apricot, sliced

¼ cup water

Preparation:

Rinse the cranberries under cold running water using a large colander. Drain and fill the measuring cup. Reserve the rest for later.

Cut the top and peel the pineapple. Chop into small chunks and fill the measuring cup. Reserve the rest in the refrigerator for some other juice.

Wash the apple and cut in half. Remove the core and cut into bite-sized pieces. Set aside.

Wash the apricot and cut in half. Remove the pit and chop into small pieces. Set aside.

Now, combine cranberries, pineapple, apple, and apricot in a juicer. Process until well juiced. Transfer to serving glasses and stir in the water.

Serve immediately.

Nutrition information per serving: Kcal: 248, Protein: 4.3g, Carbs: 76.1g, Fats: 1.3g

20.   Cucumber Maple Juice

Ingredients:

1 medium-sized cucumber, sliced

2 tsp maple syrup

1 cup strawberries, chopped

1 cup spinach, torn

2 oz water

Preparation:

Wash the cucumber and cut into thin slices.

Wash the strawberries and remove the stems. Cut into bite-sized pieces and set aside.

Wash the spinach thoroughly under cold running water. Slightly drain and torn into small pieces. Set aside.

Now, combine cucumber, strawberries, and spinach in a juicer and process until juiced. Transfer to a serving glass and stir in the water and maple syrup.

Refrigerate for 5 minutes before serving.

Enjoy!

Nutrition information per serving: Kcal: 83, Protein: 6.9g, Carbs: 24.6g, Fats: 1.3g

21.   Blackberry Plum Juice

Ingredients:

1 cup fresh blackberries

1 cup plums, halved

1 cup turnip greens, chopped

½ tsp ginger, ground

1 tsp agave nectar

½ cup water

Preparation:

Wash the blackberries under cold running water. Set aside.

Wash the plums and cut in half. Remove the pits and set aside.

Rinse the turnip greens and torn with hands. Set aside.

Now, combine blackberries, plums, and turnip greens in a juicer. Process until juiced. Transfer to a serving glass and stir in the agave, ginger, and water.

Refrigerate for 5 minutes before serving.

Enjoy!

Nutrition information per serving: Kcal: 141, Protein: 4.2g, Carbs: 40.3g, Fats: 1.4g

22.   Cranberry Leek Juice

Ingredients:

1 cup fresh cranberries

1 cup leek, chopped

2 cups cherries, pitted

2 tbsp fresh mint, finely chopped

¼ cup coconut water

Preparation:

Rinse the cranberries and cherries under cold running water using a colander. Drain and set aside.

Rinse the leek and chop into small pieces. Set aside.

Cut the cherries into halves. Remove the pits and set aside.

Combine cranberries, leek, cherries, and mint in a juicer and process until juiced. Transfer to serving glasses and stir in the coconut water.

Add some ice and serve!

Nutrition information per serving: Kcal: 252, Protein: 5.3g, Carbs: 79.5g, Fats: 1.8g

23.   Peach Lettuce Juice

Ingredients:

1 large peach, chopped

1 cup of Iceberg lettuce, torn

2 large Red Delicious apples

1 large carrot, sliced

½ cup coconut water

½ lemon, peeled

Preparation:

Wash the peach and cut in half. Remove the pit and chop into small pieces. Set aside.

Rinse the lettuce thoroughly and torn with hands. Set aside.

Wash the apples and cut in half. Remove the core and cut into bite-sized pieces. Set aside.

Wash the carrot and cut into thick slices. Set aside.

Peel the lemon and cut lengthwise in half. Reserve the rest for later.

Now, combine peach, lettuce, apples, carrot, and lemon in a juicer and process until juiced.

Transfer to serving glasses and refrigerate for 5 minutes before serving.

Nutrition information per serving: Kcal: 263, Protein: 5.1g, Carbs: 84.5g, Fats: 1.2g

24.   Green Kiwi Apple Juice

Ingredients:

2 large kiwis, peeled

1 medium-sized Honeycrisp apple, cored

1 cup of fresh spinach

1 large cucumber, sliced

¼ tsp ginger powder

Preparation:

Peel the kiwis and cut lengthwise in half. Set aside.

Wash the apple and remove the core. Cut into bite-sized pieces and set aside.

Wash the spinach thoroughly and torn with hands. Place in a pot of boiling water and let it soak for 5 minutes, or until wilted. Set aside.

Wash the cucumber and cut into thick slices. Set aside.

Peel the ginger root slice and set aside.

Combine kiwis, apple, cucumber, and soaked spinach in a juicer. Process until well juiced. Transfer to a serving glass and add some ice before serving.

Nutrition information per serving: Kcal: 201, Protein: 13.2g, Carbs: 56.5g, Fats: 2.6g

25.   Melon Agave Juice

Ingredients:

1 cup of watermelon, seeded

2 tsp agave nectar

1 cup blueberries

1 cup raspberries

1 cup cranberries

1 whole lime, peeled

Preparation:

Cut the watermelon lengthwise. Cut one large wedge. Peel and cut into chunks. Remove the seeds and set aside. Reserve the rest of the melon in the refrigerator

Combine blueberries, raspberries, and cranberries in a colander and rinse under cold running water. Drain and set aside.

Peel the lime and cut lengthwise in half. Set aside.

Now, combine watermelon, blueberries, raspberries, cranberries, and lemon in a juicer. Process until juiced. Transfer to serving glasses and stir in the agave nectar.

Add some ice cubes before serving.

Enjoy!

Nutrition information per serving: Kcal: 229, Protein: 4.1g, Carbs: 54.3g, Fats: 1.6g

26.   Cherry Apple Juice

Ingredients:

1 cup fresh cherries, pitted

2 large red apples, cored

1 large banana, chopped

1 cup watercress

A handful of fresh spinach

Preparation:

Rinse the cherries under cold running water. Drain and cut in half. Remove the pits and set aside.

Wash the apple and cut in half. Remove the core and chop into small pieces. Set aside.

Peel the banana and cut into small chunks. Set aside.

Combine watercress and spinach in a colander and wash thoroughly. Torn with hands and set aside.

Now, combine cherries, apples, banana, watercress, and spinach in a juicer and process until juiced.

Transfer to serving glasses and add few ice cubes before serving.

Enjoy!

Nutrition information per serving: Kcal: 390, Protein: 6.6g, Carbs: 113g, Fats: 1.7g

27.   Grape Pear Juice

Ingredients:

1 cup green grapes

1 large pear, cored

1 medium-sized lemon, peeled

2 large cucumbers, sliced

Preparation:

Rinse the green grapes under cold running water. Drain and remove the stems. Fill the measuring cup and set aside.

Rinse the pear and remove the core. Cut into bite-sized pieces and set aside.

Peel the lemon and cut into quarters. Set aside.

Wash the cucumbers and cut into thin slices. Set aside.

Now, combine grapes, pear, lemon, and cucumber in a juicer. Process until juiced. Transfer to serving glasses and stir well.

Refrigerate for 5-10 minutes before serving.

Enjoy!

Nutrition information per serving: Kcal: 119, Protein: 18.6g, Carbs: 32.2g, Fats: 0.2g

28.   Lime Carrot Juice

Ingredients:

3 large carrots, sliced

1 large lime, peeled

½ cup cucumber, sliced

1 large pear, cored

¼ cup fresh mint

½ cup broccoli, chopped

¼ tsp ginger powder

2 oz water

Preparation:

Wash and peel the carrots. Remove the tops and cut into thin slices.

Peel the lime and cut into quarters. Set aside.

Peel the cucumber and chop into small pieces. Fill the measuring cup and reserve the rest in the refrigerator. Set aside.

Wash the pear and remove the core. Cut into bite-sized pieces and set aside.

Combine broccoli and mint in a large colander. Rinse under cold running water. Drain and set aside.

Now, combine carrots, lime, cucumber, pear, mint, broccoli, and ginger powder in a juicer. Process until juiced.

Transfer to serving glasses and stir in the water

Refrigerate for 10 minutes before serving.

Nutrition information per serving: Kcal: 141, Protein: 5.5g, Carbs: 45.7g, Fats: 0.9g

29.   Carrot Fuji Juice

Ingredients:

1 cup fresh strawberries, chopped

1 large carrot, sliced

1 medium-sized Fuji apple, cored and chopped

1 medium-sized orange, peeled and wedged

1 cup cucumber, sliced

Preparation:

Wash the carrot and cut into thin slices. Set aside.

Wash the apple and cut in half. Remove the core and cut into bite-sized pieces. Set aside.

Wash the strawberries and remove the top stems. Cut into small pieces and set aside.

Peel the orange and divide into wedges. Set aside.

Wash the cucumber and cut into thin slices. Set aside.

Combine carrots, apple, strawberries, orange, and cucumber in a juicer. Process until juiced. Transfer to the serving glasses refrigerate for 5-10 minutes before serving.

Enjoy!

Nutrition information per serving: Kcal: 104, Protein: 3.9g, Carbs: 31.2g, Fats: 1.1g

30. Apple Vanilla Juice

Ingredients:

1 large Granny Smith's apple, cored and chopped

1 large lemon, peeled

1 large cucumber, sliced

¼ tsp vanilla extract

Preparation:

Wash the apple and remove the core. Cut into bite-sized pieces and set aside.

Peel the lemon and cut into quarters. Set aside.

Wash the cucumber and cut into thick slices. Set aside.

Wash the fresh mint and soak in water for 5 minutes.

Now, combine apple, lemon, cucumber, and mint in a juicer and process until juiced.

Transfer to serving glasses and stir in the peppermint extract.

Garnish with some extra mint leaves and add some ice before serving.

Enjoy!

Nutrition information per serving: Kcal: 170, Protein: 2.3g, Carbs: 22.3g, Fats: 1.4g

31.   Kiwi Watermelon Juice

Ingredients:

1 large kiwi, peeled

2 cups watermelon, chopped

1 cup raspberries

1 large orange, peeled

2 oz coconut water

Preparation:

Peel the kiwi and cut lengthwise in half. Set aside.

Cut the watermelon lengthwise. For two cups, you will need about two large wedges. Peel and cut into chunks. Remove the seeds and set aside. Reserve the rest of the melon for some other juices. Set aside.

Rinse the raspberries thoroughly under cold running water. Drain and set aside.

Peel the orange and divide into wedges. Set aside.

Now, combine kiwi, watermelon, raspberries, and orange in a juicer. Process until juiced and transfer to serving glasses. Stir in the coconut water and refrigerate for a while before serving.

Enjoy!

Nutrition information per serving: Kcal: 232, Protein: 5.8g, Carbs: 71.4g, Fats: 1.8g

32. Pineapple Mint Juice

Ingredients:

1 cup pineapple, chopped

1 tbsp fresh mint, chopped

2 large limes, peeled

1 cup guava, chopped

1 large cucumber, sliced

Preparation:

Peel the limes and cut lengthwise in half. Set aside.

Wash the guava and cut into bite-sized pieces. Fill the measuring cup and reserve the rest for some other recipe in a refrigerator.

Cut the top of a pineapple and peel it using a sharp knife. Cut into bite-sized pieces and fill the measuring cup. Reserve the rest of the pineapple in a refrigerator.

Wash the cucumber and cut into thin slices. Set aside.

Place chopped mint into a small bowl and add 3 tbsp of boiling water. Let it sit for 5 minutes.

Now, combine pineapple, limes, guava, and cucumber in a juicer. Process until well juiced and transfer to serving glasses. Drain the mint water and add to juice. Refrigerate for 10-15 minutes before serving.

Nutrition information per serving: Kcal: 158, Protein: 4.7g, Carbs: 47.9g, Fats: 1.1g

33.   Cucumber Plum Juice

Ingredients:

1 large cucumber, sliced

5 whole plums, pitted

1 cup blackberries

3 small strawberries, chopped

1 cup Romaine lettuce, chopped

2 oz water

Preparation:

Wash the cucumber and cut into thin slices. Set aside.

Wash the plums and cut in half. Remove the pits and cut into quarters. Set aside.

Wash the blackberries under cold running water using a colander. Slightly drain and set aside.

Wash the strawberries and remove the stems. Cut into halves and set aside.

Rinse the lettuce thoroughly under cold running water. Drain and roughly chop it. Set aside.

Now, combine cucumber, plums, blackberries, strawberries, and lettuce in a juicer and process until juice. Transfer to serving glasses and stir in the water.

Refrigerate for 10 minutes before serving.

Nutrition information per serving: Kcal: 221, Protein: 7.5g, Carbs: 69.1g, Fats: 2.1g

34. Pomegranate Carrot Juice

Ingredients:

1 cup pomegranate seeds

1 large carrot, peeled

1 large lemon, peeled

1 large apricot, pitted

1 large orange, wedged

2 oz coconut water

Preparation:

Cut the top of the pomegranate fruit using a sharp knife. Slice down to each of the white membranes inside of the fruit. Pop the seeds into measuring cup and set aside.

Peel and wash the carrot. Cut into thin slices and set aside.

Peel the lemon and cut lengthwise in half. Set aside.

Wash the apricot and cut in half. Remove the pit and cut into small pieces. Set aside.

Peel the orange and divide into wedges. Set aside.

Combine pomegranate seeds, carrot, lemon, apricot, and orange in a juicer. Process until well juiced and transfer to serving glasses. Stir in the coconut water and add few ice cubes before serving.

Nutrition information per serving: Kcal: 241, Protein: 7.3g, Carbs: 73.9g, Fats: 2.3g

35.   Peach Kiwi Juice

Ingredients:

2 large peaches, pitted

1 large kiwi, peeled

1 large Fuji apple, cored and chopped

1 large orange, peeled

1 cup strawberries, chopped

1 large lemon, peeled

2 oz water

Preparation:

Wash the peaches and cut in half. Remove the pits and cut into small pieces. Set aside.

Peel the kiwi and lemon. Cut lengthwise into halves and set aside.

Wash the apple and cut in half. Remove the core and cut into bite-sized pieces. Set aside.

Peel the orange and divide into wedges. Cut each wedge in half and set aside.

Wash the strawberries under cold running water. Remove the green parts and cut into bite-sized pieces. Set aside.

Combine peaches, kiwi, lemon, apple, orange, and strawberries in a juicer. Process until well juiced. Transfer to serving glasses and stir in the water. Add some ice and serve.

Enjoy!

Nutrition information per serving: Kcal: 345, Protein: 7.8g, Carbs: 105g, Fats: 2.3g

36.   Pomegranate Apple Juice

Ingredients:

1 cup of pomegranate seeds

1 large green apple, cored

1 cup cranberries

4 whole plums, pitted and chopped

1 tsp maple syrup

Preparation:

Cut the top of the pomegranate fruit using a sharp knife. Slice down to each of the white membranes inside of the fruit. Pop the seeds into a measuring cup and set aside.

Wash the apple and cut in half. Remove the core and cut into bite-sized pieces. Set aside.

Wash the cranberries thoroughly and drain. Set aside.

Wash the plums and cut in half. Remove the pits and cut into bite-sized pieces. Set aside.

Now, combine pomegranate, apple, cranberries, and plums in a juicer. Process until well juiced. Transfer to a serving glass and stir in the maple syrup. Optionally, add some ice before serving.

Enjoy!

Nutrition information per serving: Kcal: 264, Protein: 4.5g, Carbs: 78.6g, Fats: 1.1g

37. Sour Spinach Lemon Juice

Ingredients:

1 cup fresh spinach, chopped

1 whole lemon, peeled

1 cup cranberries

1 cup beet greens, chopped

½ cup water

Preparation:

Wash the baby spinach thoroughly and torn it with hands.

Peel the lemon and cut lengthwise. Set aside.

Place the cranberries in a colander and wash under cold running water. Drain and set aside.

Rinse the beet greens under running water using a colander. Roughly chop it using hands and set aside.

Combine spinach, lemon, cranberries, and turnip greens in a juicer. Process until juiced. Transfer to serving glasses and stir in the water.

Add some ice and serve immediately.

Nutritional information per serving: Kcal: 51, Protein: 4.3g, Carbs: 23.6g, Fats: 0.4g

38.   Sweet Strawberry Juice

Ingredients:

1 cup of strawberries, chopped

1 large Granny Smith's apple, cored

1 cup cranberries

1 large carrot, sliced

1 whole lemon, peeled

1 large orange, peeled and wedged

1 tsp stevia powder

Preparation:

Place the strawberries and cranberries in a colander and wash under cold running water. Drain and cut in half. Set aside.

Wash the apple and remove the core. Cut into bite-sized pieces and set aside.

Wash the carrot and cut into thick slices. Set aside.

Peel the lemon cut lengthwise in half. Set aside.

Peel the orange and divide into wedges. Set aside.

Combine apple, cranberries, strawberries, carrots, lemon, and orange in juicer and process until juiced. Transfer to serving glasses and stir in the water and stevia powder.

Add few ice cubes, or refrigerate for a while minutes before serving.

Nutritional information per serving: Kcal: 268, Protein: 5.6g, Carbs: 89.1g, Fats: 1.6g

39. Squash Orange Juice

Ingredients:

2 cups butternut squash, chopped

1 large orange, peeled and wedged

1 cup pomegranate seeds

1 whole lemon, peeled

1 cup celery, chopped

2 oz water

Preparation:

Peel the butternut squash and remove the seeds using a spoon. Cut into small cubes and reserve the rest of the squash for some other recipe. Wrap in a plastic foil and refrigerate.

Peel the orange and lemon. Divide orange into wedges and cut lemon lengthwise in half. Set aside.

Wash the celery and chop into small pieces. Set aside.

Cut the top of the pomegranate fruit using a sharp knife. Slice down to each of the white membranes inside of the fruit. Pop the seeds into a medium bowl.

Now, combine butternut squash, orange, pomegranate seeds, lemon, and celery in a juicer and process until juiced.

Transfer to serving glasses and stir in the water. Add few ice cubes and serve.

Enjoy!

Nutritional information per serving: Kcal: 251, Protein: 7.3g, Carbs: 79g, Fats: 1.8g

40.   Grapefruit Cucumber Juice

Ingredients:

1 large grapefruit, peeled and wedged

1 large cucumber, sliced

1 cup papaya, chopped

1 small Red Delicious apple, cored and chopped

2 oz coconut water

1 tsp maple syrup

Preparation:

Peel the grapefruit and divide into wedges. Set aside.

Wash the cucumber and cut into thick slices. Set aside.

Peel the papaya and cut lengthwise in half. Scoop out the black seeds and flesh using a spoon. Cut into small chunks and fill the measuring cup. Reserve the rest for some other juice. Set aside.

Wash the apple and remove the core. Cut into bite-sized pieces and set aside.

Combine grapefruit, cucumber, papaya, and apple in a juicer. Transfer to serving glasses and stir in the coconut water and maple syrup.

Add few ice cubes and serve immediately.

Nutritional information per serving: Kcal: 264, Protein: 5.1g, Carbs: 76.9g, Fats: 1.3g

41.   Fuji Orange Juice

Ingredients:

1 small Fuji apple, cored

1 large carrot, sliced

1 large orange, peeled and wedged

1 cup cherries, halved and pitted

1 whole lemon, peeled

2 oz water

Preparation:

Wash the apple and remove the core. Cut into bite-sized pieces and set aside.

Peel the orange and lemon. Divide orange into wedges and cut lemon lengthwise in half. Set aside.

Wash the carrot and cut into thick slices. Set aside.

Wash the cherries thoroughly and cut into halves. Remove the pits and set aside.

Now, combine apple, orange, carrot, lemon, cherries in a juicer and process until juiced. Transfer to serving glasses and add some ice before serving.

Enjoy!

Nutritional information per serving: Kcal: 253, Protein: 5.3g, Carbs: 78.2g, Fats: 1.1g

42.   Kiwi Maple Juice

Ingredients:

2 large kiwis, peeled

1 large lemon, peeled

1 cup pineapple, chunked

1 large carrot, sliced

1 large yellow apple, cored

1 tsp maple syrup

Preparation:

Peel the kiwis and lemon. Cut lengthwise into halves and set aside.

Cut the top of a pineapple and peel it using a sharp knife. Cut into small chunks and fill the measuring cup. Reserve the rest of the pineapple in a refrigerator.

Wash the carrot and cut into thick slices. Set aside.

Wash the apple and remove the core. Cut into bite-sized pieces and set aside.

Now, combine kiwis, lemon, pineapple, carrot, and apple in a juicer. Transfer to serving glasses and stir in the maple syrup. Optionally, add some ice before serving.

Nutritional information per serving: Kcal: 132, Protein: 8.9g, Carbs: 35.4g, Fats: 1.7g

43.　　Coconut Watermelon Juice

Ingredients:

1 cup watermelon, seeded and chopped

1 cup mango, chopped

1 large Granny Smith's apple, cored

1 cup black grapes, stems removed

2 oz fresh coconut water

Preparation:

Cut the watermelon lengthwise. For one cup, you will need about 1 large wedge. Peel and cut into chunks. Remove the seeds and set aside. Reserve the rest for some other juice.

Wash the mango and cut into chunks. Set aside.

Wash the apple and remove the core. Cut into bite-sized pieces and set aside.

Wash the green grapes using a colander and set aside.

Now, combine grapes, watermelon, mango, and apple in a juicer and process until juiced.

Transfer to serving glasses and stir in the coconut water. Add few ice cubes or refrigerate before serving.

Enjoy!

Nutritional information per serving: Kcal: 288, Protein: 3.7g, Carbs: 80g, Fats: 1.5g

44.   Sour Cherry Grape Juice

Ingredients:

1 cup sour cherries, pitted

2 cups green grapes

1 small banana, peeled

1 whole lime, peeled

1 tbsp coconut water

Preparation:

Rinse the cherries using a colander. Drain and cut each in half. Remove the pits and fill the measuring cup. Reserve the rest in the refrigerator.

Rinse the grapes under cold running water and remove the stems. Set aside.

Peel the banana and cut into chunks. Set aside.

Peel the lime and cut lengthwise in half. Set aside.

Now, combine cherries, grapes, banana, and lime in a juicer and process until juiced. Transfer to a serving glass and stir in the coconut water.

Serve immediately.

Nutrition information per serving: Kcal: 292, Protein: 4.1g, Carbs: 82.9g, Fats: 1.3g

45.   Cucumber Pomegranate Juice

Ingredients:

1 cup cucumber, sliced

½ cup pomegranate seeds

1 cup pumpkin, cubed

1 whole lemon, peeled

1 cup broccoli, chopped

Preparation:

Wash the cucumber and cut into thin slices. Fill the measuring cup and reserve the rest in the refrigerator. Set aside.

Cut the top of the pomegranate fruit using a sharp knife. Slice down to each of the white membranes inside of the fruit. Pop the seeds into a measuring cup and reserve the rest in the refrigerator for some other recipe.

Cut the top of a pumpkin. Cut lengthwise in half and then scrape out the seeds. Cut one large wedge and peel it. Cut into small cubes and fill the measuring cup. Reserve the rest in the refrigerator.

Peel the lemon and cut lengthwise in half. Set aside.

Wash the broccoli and trim off the outer leaves. Cut into bite-sized pieces and fill the measuring cup. Reserve the rest for later.

Trim off the outer wilted layers of the fennel. Roughly chop it and fill the measuring cup. Reserve the rest for later.

Now, combine cucumber, pomegranate seeds, pumpkin, lemon, and broccoli in a juicer and process until well juiced. Transfer to a serving glass and optionally, add some honey or agave nectar for a sweet taste.

Add some crushed ice and serve.

Nutrition information per serving: Kcal: 210, Protein: 3.9g, Carbs: 63.7g, Fats: 2.3g

46.   Mango Mint Juice

Ingredients:

1 cup mango, chunked

1 cup fresh mint, torn

1 small Golden Delicious apple, cored

1 medium-sized peach, pitted

2 medium-sized strawberries, chopped

Preparation:

Peel the mango and cut into small chunks. Fill the measuring cup and reserve the rest in the refrigerator.

Rinse the mint thoroughly under cold running water and torn with hands. Set aside. You can soak mint in hot water for 2 minutes, but it's optional.

Wash the apple and cut lengthwise in half. Remove the core and cut into bite-sized pieces. Set aside.

Wash the peach and cut in half. Remove the pit and cut into small pieces. Set aside.

Wash the strawberries and remove the stems. Cut into small pieces and set aside.

Now, combine mint, apple, mango, peach, and strawberries in a juicer and process until well juiced. Transfer to a serving glass and add few ice cubes.

Serve immediately.

Nutrition information per serving: Kcal: 227, Protein: 4.1g, Carbs: 64.9g, Fats: 1.6g

47.   Cranberry Sage Juice

Ingredients:

1 cup cranberries

1 cup cucumber, sliced

1 large honeydew melon wedge

2 large strawberries, chopped

1 oz coconut water

2 tsp fresh sage, finely chopped

Preparation:

Wash the cucumber and cut into thin slices. Fill the measuring cup and reserve the rest for later. Set aside.

Using a small colander, rinse well the cranberries. Drain and set aside.

Cut melon lengthwise in half. Scoop out the seeds and then wash the melon. Cut one wedge and peel it. Cut into bite-sized pieces and set aside.

Wash the strawberries and remove the stems. Chop into small pieces and set aside.

Now, combine cranberries, cucumber melon, and strawberries in a juicer. Process until well juiced. Transfer to a serving glass and stir in the coconut water and sage.

Serve immediately.

Nutrition information per serving: Kcal: 96, Protein: 1.8g, Carbs: 31.4g, Fats: 0.6g

48. Banana Plum Juice

Ingredients:

1 cup banana, chunked

2 whole plums, chopped

1 cup strawberries, chopped

1 cup cantaloupe, chopped

¼ tsp cinnamon, ground

Preparation:

Peel the banana and cut into chunks. Fill the measuring cup and reserve the rest. Set aside.

Wash the plums and cut each in half. Remove the pits and cut into small pieces. Set aside.

Wash the strawberries and remove the stems. Cut into bite-sized pieces and set aside.

Cut the cantaloupe in half. Scrape out the seeds and cut one large wedge. Peel and chop into small pieces and fill the measuring cup. Wrap the rest in a plastic foil and refrigerate for later.

Now, combine banana, plums, strawberries, and cantaloupe in a juicer and process until juiced. Transfer to a serving glass and stir in the cinnamon.

Add some crushed ice and serve immediately.

Nutrition information per serving: Kcal: 249, Protein: 4.8g, Carbs: 73.1g, Fats: 1.5g

49.   Black Grape Blueberry Juice

Ingredients:

1 cup fresh blackberries

1 cup black grapes, stems removed

1 cup fresh strawberries

1 medium-sized Fuji apple, cored

2 oz coconut water

Preparation:

Combine blackberries and strawberries in a colander. Wash under cold running water and set aside.

Rinse the grapes well and set aside.

Wash the apple and remove the core. Cut into bite-sized pieces and set aside.

Now, process blackberries, grapes, strawberries, and apple in a juicer. Transfer to serving glasses and stir in the coconut water.

Optionally, add some ice cubes before serving.

Nutritional information per serving: Kcal: 201, Protein: 4.3g, Carbs: 63.4g, Fats: 1.7g

50.   Strawberry Mint Juice

Ingredients:

1 cup frozen strawberries, chopped

1 cup fresh mint, torn

2 medium-sized red apples, cored

1 large honeydew melon wedge

2 oz coconut water

Preparation:

Chop the strawberries into halves or smaller pieces. Set aside.

Wash the mint thoroughly and torn with hands. Set aside.

Wash the apples and remove the core. Cut into bite-sized pieces. Set aside.

Cut the honeydew melon lengthwise in half. Scoop out the seeds using a spoon. Cut and peel 2 large wedges. Cut into small chunks and place in a bowl. Wrap the rest of the melon in a plastic foil and refrigerate.

Now, combine strawberries, mint, apple, and melon chops in a juicer. Process until juiced.

Transfer to serving glasses and stir in the coconut water.

Add ice cubes and serve immediately.

Nutritional information per serving: Kcal: 293, Protein: 4.5g, Carbs: 84g, Fats: 1.6g

51.   Salted Green Celery Juice

Ingredients:

1 cup fresh celery, chopped

1 cup fresh kale, chopped

3 large leeks, chopped

2 cups beet greens, trimmed

1 large cucumber

1 ginger knob, sliced

½ tsp Himalayan salt

Preparation:

In a large colander, combine celery, leek, beet greens, and kale. Rinse thoroughly under cold running water and drain. Chop all into small pieces and set aside.

Wash the cucumber and cut into thick slices. Set aside.

Peel the ginger and set aside.

Combine celery, leek, beet greens, kale, cucumber, and ginger in a juicer. Process until well juiced.

Transfer to serving glasses and stir in the salt.

Refrigerate for 10 minutes before serving.

Nutritional information per serving: Kcal: 230, Protein: 11.5g, Carbs: 63.2g, Fats: 2.1g

52. Sweet Carrot Juice

Ingredients:

1 large carrot, sliced

1 cup apricots, pitted and halved

1 large lemon, peeled

1 medium-sized Granny Smith's apple, cored and chopped

1 tbsp agave nectar

2 oz water

Preparation:

Wash the apricots and cut in half. Remove the pits and fill the measuring cup. Reserve the rest for some other juice. Set aside.

Peel the lemon and cut lengthwise in half. Set aside.

Wash the carrot and cut into thick slices and set aside.

Wash the apple and remove the core. Cut into bite-sized pieces and set aside.

Now, combine apricots, lemon, carrot, and apple in a juicer and process until juiced.

Transfer to serving glasses and stir in the agave nectar and water.

Refrigerate for 15 minutes before serving.

Nutrition information per serving: Kcal: 243, Protein: 4.2g, Carbs: 69.3g, Fats: 1.3g

53.   Kiwi Avocado Juice

Ingredients:

2 kiwis, peeled

½ ripe avocado, peeled and sliced

1 large cucumber

1 cup frozen strawberries

1 small lime, peeled

2 tbsp fresh mint

Preparation:

Peel the kiwis and cut into halves, then into quarters. Set aside.

Peel the avocado and cut in half. Remove the pit and cut one half into thin slices. Reserve the other half in the refrigerator.

Wash the cucumber and chop into bite-sized pieces.

Wash the strawberries and cut into halves. Set aside.

Peel the lime and cut into quarters. Set aside.

Wash the mint leaves and soak in water for 10 minutes.

Process kiwis, cucumber, strawberries, lime, and mint in a juicer until nicely juiced.

Transfer to serving glasses and serve immediately.

Nutritional information per serving: Kcal: 181, Protein: 6.2g, Carbs: 41.9g, Fats: 21.9g

54.   Orange Cantaloupe Juice

Ingredients:

2 large oranges, peeled

1 cup cantaloupe, cubed

2 medium-sized radishes, trimmed

1 ginger root knob, 1-inch

1 tbsp liquid honey

½ cup pomegranate seeds

2 oz water

Preparation:

Peel the oranges and divide into wedges. Set aside.

Cut the cantaloupe in half. Scoop out the seeds and flesh. You will need about one large wedge for one cup. Cut and peel it. Chop into chunks and set aside. Reserve the rest of the cantaloupe in a refrigerator.

Wash the radishes and trim off the green parts. Cut into small pieces and set aside.

Peel the ginger root knob and set aside.

Cut the top of the pomegranate fruit using a sharp knife. Slice down to each of the white membranes inside of the fruit. Pop the seeds into a measuring cup and set aside.

Combine oranges, cantaloupe, radishes, ginger, and pomegranate seeds in a juicer and process until juiced. Transfer to serving glasses and stir in the honey and water.

Add few ice cubes or refrigerate for 10 minutes before serving.

Nutrition information per serving: Kcal: 279, Protein: 4.9g, Carbs: 82.3g, Fats: 0.8g

55. Sweet Lemon Juice

Ingredients:

1 tbsp honey, raw

1 whole lemon, peeled

1 cup strawberries, chopped

1 whole lime, peeled

2 oz water

Preparation:

Peel the lemon and lime. Cut each fruit lengthwise in half and set aside.

Wash the strawberries and remove the stems. Cut into bite-sized pieces and set aside.

Now, combine lemon, lime, and strawberries in a juicer and process until juiced. Transfer to a serving glass and stir in the water and honey.

Refrigerate for 5 minutes before serving.

Enjoy!

Nutrition information per serving: Kcal: 81, Protein: 5.8g, Carbs: 20.8g, Fats: 1.4g

56.   Peach Mint Juice

Ingredients:

1 large peach, pitted and chopped

1 small Granny Smith's apple, cored and chopped

1 whole banana, sliced

1 oz coconut water

1 medium-sized plum, chopped

1 tbsp mint, finely chopped

¼ tsp cinnamon, ground

Preparation:

Wash the peach and cut lengthwise in half. Remove the pit and cut into bite-sized pieces. Set aside.

Wash the apple and cut in half. Remove the core and chop into small pieces. Set aside.

Peel the banana and cut into thin slices. Set aside.

Rinse the plum and cut in half. Remove the pit and chop into small pieces. Set aside.

Now, combine peach, apple, bananas, and plum in a juicer and process until well juiced. Transfer to a serving glass and stir in the cinnamon and coconut water.

Sprinkle with mint and add ice.

Enjoy!

Nutrition information per serving: Kcal: 412, Protein: 5.5g, Carbs: 124g, Fats: 1.7g

ADDITIONAL TITLES FROM THIS AUTHOR

70 Effective Meal Recipes to Prevent and Solve Being Overweight: Burn Fat Fast by Using Proper Dieting and Smart Nutrition

By

Joe Correa CSN

48 Acne Solving Meal Recipes: The Fast and Natural Path to Fixing Your Acne Problems in Less Than 10 Days!

By

Joe Correa CSN

41 Alzheimer's Preventing Meal Recipes: Reduce or Eliminate Your Alzheimer's Condition in 30 Days or Less!

By

Joe Correa CSN

70 Effective Breast Cancer Meal Recipes: Prevent and Fight Breast Cancer with Smart Nutrition and Powerful Foods

By

Joe Correa CSN

www.ingramcontent.com/pod-product-compliance
Lightning Source LLC
Chambersburg PA
CBHW030256030426
42336CB00009B/397